Negative Calorie Diet & Weight Loss

LELA GIBSON

CONTENTS

Introduction   i

Negative Calorie Diet: What Is It   2

Negative Calorie Food List   4

How To Make The Transition To Negative Calorie Diet   9

Negative Calorie Diet Recipes   15

Breakfast Recipes   16

Lunch Recipes   20

Dinner Recipes   26

Snacks   33

Negative Calorie Diet And Exercise: An Effective Way To Lose Weight Fast   40

I need your help...   47

LELA GIBSON

Negative Calorie Diet

Cookbook & Guide Which Will Help You To Burn Body Fat, Lose Weight And Live Healthy

Lela Gibson

Introduction

I would like to thank you for buying the book, "Negative Calorie Diet".

This book contains proven steps and strategies on how to burn body fat, lose weight and eat healthy.

Are you on the verge of giving up on your weight loss goals? Have you tried reducing your fat intake, eating fewer carbohydrates and all the diets that call for eating fewer proteins and carbohydrates, drank a lot of water, but you don't lose any weight? Does nothing seem to work?Well, I guess losing hope is understandable, but wait, DO NOT GIVE UP JUST YET! There is one more option, the best option in fact: The Negative Calorie Diet.

If we are to go by the facts, theNegative Calorie Diet is the fastest way to lose weight; you can lose up to 14 pounds a week when you adopt the diet! Thanks to this diet, losing weight is no longer a random dream or a hope; it is a reality for thousands of people across the globe.

In this book, you will learn more about the Negative Calorie Diet, how it works and some amazing recipes that will help you burn fat.

Thanks again for buying this book, I hope you enjoy it!

Negative Calorie Diet: What Is It

This unique diet draws upon theidea that some foodshave the 'negative calorie' effect that we ought to consider in burning fat. A food is considered to have a negative calorie effect when the calories these foods use to digest are typically higherthan the calories in the foods themselves.

When you eat something, you begin by chewing, a process that consumes energy. Some foods such as those higher in stringy fibers like celery will require more chewing, which will result in more energy expenditure, and there are otherslike pasta and cakes that don't require as much chewing.

After chewing, the foods go to the stomach through the esophagus and the other processes of digestion take over until absorption takes place and the body excretes the residual mass.

With negative calorie foods, this entire process uses up more calories than the foods have. The extra calories the body has to provide in order to process the foods are taken from the fat stores, and the more of these negative calorie foods you eat, the more your fat stores will lose calories, and as a result, the more fatyou will lose.

Let us take broccoli as an example: 100 grams (contains 25 calories).

When you eat 100 grams of broccoli, it takes your body about 80 calories worth of energy to digest it. This results in a net calorie use of 55 calories that should come from the fat stores in your body. As you can see, the 55 calories make up the negative net calorie.

Let us now take a counter example of a piece of cake containing 400 calories.

Your body will take about 150 calories to digest the piece of cake, leaving net 250 caloriesdeposited in the body and stored as fat.

The negative calorie diet consists of over 100 foods proven to have negative calorie qualities. Most of these foods are fruits and veggies that are high in fiber. Let us look at them in more detail in the following chapter.

Negative Calorie Food List

Here is a list of negative calorie foods:

Vegetables

Vegetables are highly nutritious and not high in calories when compared to many processed foods. Nonetheless, some vegetables are superior especially when it comes to the negative calorie food list. The following are vegetables you should consider including in your diet.

Artichokes	Bean sprouts	Broccoli	Cabbage	Cauliflower
Asparagus	Beets and beet greens	Brussels sprouts	Carrots	Celery
Chives	Cucumbers	Green beans	Mushrooms	Peppers (red, green, yellow)
Pumpkin	Sauerkraut	Spinach	String beans	Turnips
Corn	Eggplant	Lettuce	Peas	Pickles
Radishes	Scallions	Squash	Tomatoes	Zucchini
Garlic	Onion	Watercress		

Fruits

Just like vegetables, fruits are a healthier option and always the recommended healthy alternative to sugary foods. It is therefore a better idea to snack on a bunch of grapes than it is to snack on candy.

However, when it comes to fruit choices, you also need to make better choices because some fruits are high in calories; thus, not providing you the negative calorie effect you are looking for in negative calorie foods

The list below contains some good negative-calorie fruits you can eat:

Apples	Blackberries	Cantaloupe	Cranberries	Grapefruit
Honeydew melon	Lemons	Mangoes	Apricots	Blueberries
Cherries	Currants	Grapes	Kiwi	Limes
Nectarines	Oranges	Pears	Pomegranates	Strawberries
Watermelon	Peaches	Pineapple	Raspberries	Tangerines
Prunes				

Herbs and Spices

When it is a question of what you eat, even herbs and spices matter. Below is a complete list of herbs and spices you should always go for.

Chili pepper	Cloves	Ginger	Parsley	Cinnamon
Mustard seeds	Cayenne	Anise	Coriander/ Cilantro	Dill
Cumin	Fennel seeds			

You can take various opportunities to add herbs and spices to your food. You can use them whenever you cook and you can add them to your soups and salads. Various herbs and spices can add different flavors to your food. Therefore, you should make it a point to experiment with them.

Meat, Fish and Seafood

Red meat can be harmful to you, and many negative calorie diets don't recommend it; however, you do not have to avoid eating meat altogether, as it provides essential proteins and other nutrients. A good source of protein is fish for instance. Fish is lower in calories but high in essential nutrients like omega-3 fatty acids.

If you are allergic to fish, or if you are not a big fan of it, you can alternatively include small/reasonable potions of meat and chicken in your diet (I will teach you how in the recipes section).

The table below shows some of the best fish and seafood to include in your diet:

Clams	Crayfish	Mussels	Shrimp	Crab
Flounder	Tuna	Abalone	Buffalo fish	Cod
Terrapin	Bass	Catfish	Trout	

How To Make The Transition To Negative Calorie Diet

Now that you know what to eat, let us see exactly how you are going to be eating all that.

1. Make a smooth transition into the negative calorie diet so that you are comfortable with the entire process. Start by adding some negative calorie foods to the foods you normally eat in every meal in the 1:1 ratio. For instance, if having pasta with meatballs, you can serve 50% of this food and add chunks of zucchini to fill the other half.

You can also add a mixed salad to each meal you have; the salad should comprise of not less than 90% negative calorie foods. This means you have to look for ways to substitute any unwanted content such as any creamy high-fat substances with something like raspberry vinaigrette.

After some time, start slowly substituting the foods with the good (negative calorie) ones until your plate contains up to 90% negative calorie foods.

Note: We are only adding vegetables and fruits so far, not necessarily fully prepared negative calorie meals. Next, we will discuss the recipes so that you have entirely cooked meals too.

2.Use several vegetables to make a stir-fry. You can also make smoothie shakes with your favorite fruits including some berries. However, you need to be careful when drinking smoothies. Remember, smoothies are mostly drank, not chewed. This means you won't be burning any calories from the action of chewing. Thus, you should keep your smoothie consumption to a minimum. Also, use more negative calorie vegetables than fruits whenever you make smoothies.

As said before, the negative calorie diet is largely a fruits and vegetables diet. However, this does not mean you should now start worrying about how you will survive as a vegetarian.

You can occasionallyenjoy small servings of chicken and some meat, and the recipes in the following chapter will reflect that. Nonetheless, the meats have to be in small amounts; remember, you are losing weight and so, you have to make some sacrifices.

First Thing to Do

Buy all the foods you think you require from the list, wash, cut them into bits then seal them in airtight containers for storage (in the fridge) so that you will have them handy anytime you need them. You do not want to come home from work tired in the evening without having a bunch of these foods readily available. If you do, you will be extremely tempted to grab something unhealthy.

If you are wondering whether you will be hungry on this diet plan, just know that you will not because these foods are filling because they are high in fiber as well as water; the perfect combination to be full.

Buying the foods you need is not enough. You also need to get rid of the foods you don't need to eat. As you will be easing into the diet, you can go about getting rid of such foods a little at a time. However, in the end, your pantry and your refrigerator should only contain the negative calorie foods.

Note: While on this diet, you should have no room for alcohol, sugar, or any sugar substitutes except stevia simply because sugar intake causes your body to produce more insulin. This hormone signals/tells the fat cells to pick up and convert any excess glucose into fat. Therefore, eating more sugar means more production of insulin and consequently, more deposits in the fat cells. We are trying to reduce fat in your body, not create more of it. In this regard, avoid all commercial dressings since most of them contain sugar and high fat content.

Now that we have that out of the way, let us start cooking!

Second Thing to Do

Once you have identified the foods you want to eat, the next step is to actually get rid of the foods you want to stay away from. Let's face it, many times you end up eating some foods, not because you're hungry, but simply because you've seen them. High calorie foods often tend to be appetizing and inviting. Macronutrients such as carbohydrates work to stimulate the brain's pleasure center. This means you end up craving high carb foods and overeating in order to keep getting that 'comfort' they provide. Unfortunately, such foods are quite high in calories. Therefore, they ensure that your body has more than enough calories to store up. This is why you need to do a kitchen sweep.

Start by checking your list and determining which foods need to go. If you've not fully transitioned to the negative calorie diet, you need to determine which foods you'll get rid of first and which ones you'll get rid of later. Write down a list so that you can check your progress. For example, you may start by getting rid of pasta and red meat. Next, you can get rid of alcoholic drinks and high calorie fruits.

The idea is to gradually get rid of those foods that are high in calories. This will leave you with foods that will help you achieve your goal on the negative calorie diet. Once you've done that, you can move on to the next step.

Note: While on this diet, you should have no room for alcohol, sugar, or any sugar substitutes except stevia simply because sugar intake causes your body to produce more insulin. This hormone signals/tells the fat cells to pick up and convert any excess glucose into fat. Therefore, eating more sugar means more production of insulin and consequently, more deposits in the fat cells. We are trying to reduce fat in your body, not create more of it. In this regard, avoid all commercial dressings since most of them contain sugar and high fat content.

Third Thing to Do

It's well and good to know which foods to eat when you're on the negative calorie diet but it's another thing to make a meal out of the various foods. This is why the third step is to embrace meal planning.

You can plan for breakfast, lunch, dinner and snacks. Start by asking yourself what you want to eat during such meals. For example, you may plan to eat salads for lunch. As you have read, you can actually include many negative calorie foods in salads. This means that you can create various types of salads to eat throughout the week. Take some time to think of the combinations of foods you'd want to eat. This will keep the diet fresh and interesting.

Meal planning also enables you to know what foods to buy for the week. Remember, you'll be eating a lot of fruits and vegetables. These types of foods tend to taste better when they are fresh. Unfortunately, they also tend to go bad fast. This means you'll have to plan your shopping well in order to get the best out of the foods. If you know what you'll be eating, you'll purchase whatever is needed and this will enhance your experience as you continue your diet.

Now that we have that out of the way, let us start cooking!

Negative Calorie Diet Recipes

While on a strict diet (such as this one), you might have a problem trying to decide what kind of dressing to use for your meals. Since I know it is important to be careful about what you are using, I will start by giving you two simple dressings that you will use on any meal you want.

Garlic and Herbs Dressing

Mix 1/2 cup of cold-pressed extra-virgin olive oil with juice from 1 lemon, 2 crushed garlic cloves and ¼ cup apple cider vinegar. Add some of your favorite negative caloriedried herbs such as parsley and cilantro.

This will yield 1 cup of dressing. Store the dressing in the fridge (for up to one month) to use on your foods.

Dijon and Yoghurt Dressing

For a delicious vegetable dip, mix Dijon mustard (2 tablespoons) with 2 cups low-fat yoghurt then add a pinch of chili pepper and a teaspoon of mixed dried herbs to spice it up.

Breakfast Recipes

Pumpkin Pancakes

Serves 4

Ingredients

1 cup of canned pumpkin

1 1/4 cups of water

2 teaspoons of cinnamon

2 cups Krusteaz pancake mix

1 egg, slightly beaten

1 teaspoon of baking powder

For the topping

1/4 cup of sliced pecans

5 tablespoons of pure maple syrup

Instructions

Combine all the ingredients for the pancake batter.

On a griddle or pan over medium heat sprayed with a little cooking spray, create a 10 cm circle of batter.

When the pancakes turn brown at the edges and you notice even bubbling across the top, flip them over to cook the other side.

In the meantime, toast pecans in a small pan until they turn slightly brown and give out the fragrance.

Serve with heated pure maple syrup.

Apple and Cinnamon with Almonds and Oat Bran

Serves 4

Ingredients

4 large apples

1 teaspoon of ground cinnamon

1/4 cup of oat bran

10 almonds, toasted and chopped

1 teaspoon of unrefined coconut oil

2 cups of unsweetened vanilla almond milk

2 packets monk fruit extract

Instructions

Wash the apples and cut into cubes.

Melt the coconut oil in a large nonstick skillet over medium high heat. Add the cinnamon and apples then cook for 2-3 minutes until the apples soften.

Remove from the heat, add almond milk, stir in the monk fruit extract and oat bran. Once mixed return back to the heat, stir, and bring to a simmer.

Cook for about one minute, until the mixture becomes thick and creamy.

Divide the mixture among four bowls then sprinkle each one with toasted almonds.

Negative Calorie Smoothie

Serves 2

Ingredients

5 strawberries

½ medium papaya

1 grapefruit

¼ cup ice

Instructions

Put all the ingredients in a blender; blend until smooth.

Serve and garnish with some strawberries and enjoy.

Lunch Recipes

Vegetable Soup

Serves 6

This is not your regular veggie soup; yes, it is simple, but it is full of negative calorie foods only.

Ingredients

6 cups of vegetable stock

1 cup of celery, diced

1 cup of green beans cut into about 1 inch pieces

1 medium zucchini, diced (approximately 2 cups)

1 cup small turnip, diced

1 jalapeno, seeded and finely chopped

1 medium onion, diced

1 cup of cauliflower florets

2 cups of shredded cabbage

3 cloves of garlic, finely chopped

2 cups of baby spinach

Salt and pepper to taste

Instructions

Mix the ingredients (except the spinach) in a pot, and bring to a boil.

Cover and let it simmer for 20 minutes.

Add the spinach, stir, and let it cook for one more minute.

Remove from the heat and serve.

Toast with Tomatoes

Serves 4

Ingredients

8 cups of spinach

½ ripe avocado, mashed well with a fork

Salt to taste

Freshly ground black pepper to taste

4 slices of natural gluten-free bread

4 (½-inch) slices ripe tomato

4 eggs, poached

Green hot sauce

Instructions

Place a nonstick skillet over medium high heat.

Add the spinach and cook until it wilts. Move the spinach to a colander and strain out as much water as possible. Put the now drained spinach in a bowl and season with green hot sauce and salt.

Use a toaster to toast the bread then season the avocado with salt. Evenly spreadthe pieces of avocado over each piece of toast then add a slice of tomato on top. Use pepper and salt to season the tomatoes and use the spinach mixture to top each slice evenly.

Place every piece of toast on a fresh plate. Finally, top with a poached egg and serve.

Meatballs with Mushroom Gravy

Serves 4

Ingredients

12 ounces lean ground beef

1 ounce Parmigiano Reggiano cheese, finely chopped

2 tablespoons arrowroot, dissolved in 2 teaspoons of stock

8 cups washed spinach

1 cup thinly sliced onion

4 cups sliced cremini mushrooms

Olive oil cooking spray

Freshly ground black pepper

Salt to taste

4 cups unsalted beef stock

1 cup finely chopped puffed brown rice

Instructions

Put the beef in a large bowl and push it to one side. Add rice and a cup of the stock to the other side of the mixing bowl; season with pepper and salt and allow the rice to absorb the stock for about 1 minute.

Mix the beef and rice using an electric hand mixture until well mixed. Taste and adjust the seasoning then use the mixture to form 16 meatballs.

Coat a skillet with olive oil cooking spray and place over medium heat. Once hot, put the meatballs and brown for one minute on one side. Turn and brown the opposite side for around 30 seconds and transfer to a plate.

Add the mushrooms to the skillet and sauté for a few minutes. Add the meatballs back to the skillet, then add the beef stock, arrowroot mixture, and cook until meatballs are cooked through.

Add the spinach and season with pepper and salt and cook until the spinach is wilted. Add the cheese, stir, and serve.

Dinner Recipes

Brussels Sprouts with Lemon and Almond Dressing

Serves 3-4

Ingredients

3 pints Brussels sprouts, shaved thinly

5 teaspoons of freshly minced garlic

Crushed red pepper flakes

1/2 cup of chopped fresh flat-leaf parsley

Salt

1 1/2 teaspoons of extra-virgin olive oil

1/4 cup of toasted almonds, finely chopped

1/8 teaspoon of ground cinnamon

1/2 cup freshly squeezed lemon juice

1 ounce of Parmigiano-Reggiano cheese, finely grated

Instructions

Place the Brussels in a large mixing bowl and place it aside.

Placea non-stick skillet over medium high heat then add the garlic and olive oil. Cook until the garlic turns deep golden brown. Remove from the heat then add the parsley, almonds, cinnamon, and red pepper flakes.

Return the skillet back to the heat sauté for about ten seconds.Remove from the heat, pour in the lemon juice, and then season with salt.

Add the dressing to the Brussels then toss well, add 75% of the cheese, and toss some more. Taste then add the seasoning and top with the rest of the cheese.

Chicken with Pesto

Serves 3 or 4

Ingredients

Water

6 garlic cloves, chopped

Dash of paprika

1 cup of fresh basil leaves

8 cups ofchopped escarole

Salt

1 ounce of Parmigiano-Reggiano cheese, finely grated

Olive oil cooking spray

Dash of cinnamon

Crushed red pepper flakes

1 small onion, thinly sliced

4 cups chicken stock,unsalted

12 ounces of skinless, boneless chicken breast sliced into 1/8 inch thick strips

Instructions

Pour 2 quarts of water in a medium pot and bring to a simmer. You will use this to poach the chicken.

Lightly coat a medium skillet with olive oil cooking spray then place it over medium high heat.

Add the garlic and cook until it turns golden brown. Add the cinnamon, basil leaves, red pepper flakes, onion, and paprika. Cook for roughly 2 minutes until the onion softens.

Add the escarole then cook until it is soft and wilted – for 2 more minutes. Add the stock, bring to a simmer, and then cover. Cook for about 5 minutes or until tender.

Add a pinch of salt to the simmering water and turn off the heat. Add the chicken and stir well until all parts separate. Cook until you notice the strips turning white (meaning they are half cooked). Use a slotted spoon to transfer the strips to a plate to cool.

Let the remaining mixture cook until most of the stock evaporates and looks like thick sauce or soup. Turn off the heat.

Add in half of the cheese, stir, and then season with salt to taste. Add the chicken strips then toss them to coat with the mixture and keep cooking until the strips have cooked enough through, for about 90 seconds.

Top with the remaining cheese, and then serve.

Vegetable Beef Soup

Serves 14

Note: This recipe has many ingredients and it is likely you will hate some vegetables or herbs. You can replace these vegetables and herbs with other ingredients on the negative calorie food list.

Ingredients

4 chopped onions

1 chopped red bell pepper

4 cups of sliced fresh mushrooms

10 chopped celery stalks with their leaves

2 cupsof fresh chopped broccoli

1 small chopped bunch of cilantro

5 box low sodium beef broth

1 large chopped green bell pepper

4 cups of chopped cabbage

6 large chopped fresh carrots

1 finely chopped head of garlic

6 cups of fresh chopped spinach

1 small bunch of Parsley

1 canof asparagus (drained)

2 cans of green beans (drained)

1 cupof canned artichokes (drained)

20 twists of cracked black pepper

1 tablespoon of Italian seasoning

Protein (you can use just about any meat preferably the fishes mentioned in the list)

2 10 oz. cans of tomatoes with green chili's (not drained)

2 cans of diced tomatoes with basil (not drained)

1/2 tablespoon of red pepper flakes

1 tablespoonof dried basil

2 small cans of chopped green chilies (not drained)

1 lb. 80/20 or leaner ground beef (drain if needed)

Instructions

Fill a large cooking pot halfway with the beef, chicken, or vegetable stock. Add all the canned ingredients while draining some as specified intothe pot.

Add water and all the spices then stir. Let it boil for some time, lower the heat to simmer for one hour or until the vegetables soften.

As the soup boils down, add some extra broth and stir.

Serve, garnish as desired, and enjoy.

Snacks

Apple Chips

Serves 2

Ingredients

2 large granny smith apples

1 teaspoon of stevia

1 teaspoon of cinnamon

Canola oil cooking spray

Instructions

Preheat your oven to 200 degrees.

Using a sharp knife, thinlyslice the apples crosswise. Arrange the slices on a single layer on a baking sheet then spray with canola oil cooking spray.

Evenlysprinkle the stevia and cinnamon over the apple slices.

Use the bottom third part of the oven to bake the apples until they are crisp and dry, roughly 2-2½ hours.

Alternatively, you could use a mastrad chipmaker. Not only is it easy and fast, you do not need the cooking spray. Just lay the apple slices on the chipmaker, sprinkle with cinnamon and stevia, and then microwave for 4-5 minutes.

Berry Salad

Serves 4

Ingredients

4 cups of mixed berries (blackberries, raspberries, blueberries, strawberries)

20 whole almonds, toasted and chopped

2 tablespoons of hemp hearts

1/4 cup of cooked quinoa

1 ½ tablespoons of fat free yoghurt

Instructions

Equally divide all the ingredients among four bowls and toss well to mix.

Fruit Salad

Serves 10

Ingredients

2/3 cup of fresh orange juice

1/2 teaspoon of grated lemon zest

2 cups of cubed fresh pineapple

3 kiwi fruits, peeled and sliced

2 oranges, peeled and sectioned

2 cups of blueberries

1/3 cup of fresh lemon juice

1/2 teaspoon of grated orange zest

1 teaspoon of vanilla extract

2 cups of strawberries, hulled and sliced

3 bananas, sliced

1 cup seedless grapes

Instructions

Add orange zest, orange juice, lemon juice and lemon zest, to a saucepan, place it over medium high heat, and bring to boil.

Decrease the heat to medium-low and let it simmer for 5 minutes. Remove from the heat and stir in the vanilla extract. Place it aside to cool.

Place the fruit in a clear glass bowl in layers starting with the pineapple, then strawberries, kiwi, bananas, oranges, then grapes and at the top, blueberries.

Pour the juice over the fruit layers then cover and leave in the fridge for 3-4 hours before serving.

Almond Cake with Berries

Serves 4

Ingredients

½ cup of almond meal

4 packets of monk fruit extract

1 teaspoon of vanilla extract

Olive oil cooking spray

2 eggs, separated; remove 1 yolk

3 tablespoons of raw coconut nectar

Salt

1 cup of mixed berries, mashed well with a fork

Instructions

Preheat your oven to 3750 degrees F.

Bake the almond meal until it becomes aromatic and well toasted –about 3-5 minutes. Remove from the oven and place it on a cool baking sheet.

Place the monk fruit and egg whites in a bowl and whisk until it forms stiff peaks. Use cooking spray to spray four paper cups. Using a toothpick or fork, poke holes in the bottom of each.

Place the almond meal into a mixing bowl then add the egg yolk, salt, vanilla, and coconut nectar. Fold the meringue into the mixture of almond and transfer the batter into the cups.

Place in the microwave and microwave for about thirty seconds. When the mixture has cooked through, place the cups on their sides and give them 45 seconds to cook.

Remove the cakes and place themupside down on four serving plates.

Get them off the cups and serve with berries.

Cucumber and salsa

Serves 2

Ingredients

2 cucumbers, peeled and sliced

12 garlic cloves, minced

¼ cup fresh cilantro, chopped

3 tomatoes, diced

½ sweet onion, diced

Sea salt and black pepper to taste

Instructions

Mix all ingredients except the cucumber in a bowl in order to make the salsa.

Place cucumber slices on a plate and serve with the salsa.

Negative Calorie Diet And Exercise: An Effective Way To Lose Weight Fast

I promised you some unique and cool exercise tips, right? Doing the following exercises will help you burn the fat much faster. All you have to do is to start slow and over time, increase the intensity, keep an open mind, and use the gym (for the ones that require it), where you have an instructor nearby.

Interval Training

This is all about high intensity exercises combined with short periods of rest. This will not only burn more calories than your typical cardio training, it will boost your body's ability to burn fat easily since it increases the production of the growth hormone, which is also a fat burning hormone, and adrenaline which assists in suppressing your appetite.

The intervals will work on your muscles, and help them use oxygen better so that your heart does not have to struggle to pump a lot to make them perform.

Do It!

Get on a treadmill or a stationary bike then use the guide below to start your own interval-training regimen:

Begin with a regular warm-up (any simple exercise to get your blood rushing). When done, run or pedal at a rate that is more than your regular cardio intensity by 20%. If you have never engaged in any serious cardio workouts before, you might want to check this first to understand what I am talking about.

After 30 seconds to 1 minute, reduce the intensity to a rate that is 50% less than the intensity of a regular cardio workout. Alternate the periods of 30 seconds to 1 minute of hard work with 30 seconds to 1 minute of relaxed pedaling or if you want, relaxed running for 6-10 intervals to finish your session.

As this gets simpler, increase each interval's intensity so that you work even longer during the difficult part, reduce your rest periods, or if you feel enthusiastic enough, add more intervals.

Repeat 3-4 times each week.

As you get the hang of this exercise, start the next:

Sprinting

Try sprinting up a hill since the impact on your joints will be much lower and can help you avoid injury. If there is no hilly ground in your area, try the alternative: the dag race approach. Start your sprint by increasing your speed from a jog.

To make the most of this exercise, keep the sprints short – ideally50 yards per sprint. This helps you sustain a high intensity all through and prevents injury.

If you want to increase the overall results of your sprint workout, increase your total number of sprints. This is better than going for long distance runs.

If you are new to exercising, do not do more than one workout per week. You can increase the days once you accustom to the exercise; just remember to allow at least two days of recovery between the workouts.

As you get the hang of the above exercise, start the next:

High Intensity Strength Intervals

Select two exercises that work different muscles completely or ones that use opposite movements. For instance, you can pair a pulling exercise with a pushing exercise or upper body exercise with a lower body exercise like pull-ups and squats.

For the latter, select a weight (if your instructor thinks you need one) with which you can do 10 repetitions. Alternate between the two exercises and do just five repetitions of each move in every set. Remember to rest between the sets so that you finish each set without failing.

Keep alternating between the exercises for a 10 or 15 minutes set time. Keep noting the total number of sets you can do. In subsequent sessions, try to beat your score by completing more sets in the same duration or completing the same number of sets but with heavier weights.

As you get the hang of the above exercises, start the next:

Countdown Workouts

Countdown workouts fit in the use of exercise pairs really well. They also keep you fully engaged in the exercises since you have to keep the count and pay attention.

With every round of the exercise pair, the training encompasses one lesser rep of each move; for instance, you move from a set of six to five...until zero.

You can also try density training where you pair opposing exercises for countdowns. For instance, kettlebell swing, pushups, and squat thrusts would work really well.

Do it!

Start by selecting your pair of exercises.

Perform six repetitions of the first exercise, then six reps of the other move. Go back to the first move and perform five reps then five more of the second exercise. Keep alternating until you reach zero.

In the subsequent workouts, add one rep to each exercise. If you want more countdowns, select a second pair from the list below, or just come up with your own pair of opposing moves.

Squat thrust, pushups

Kettlebell swing, squat thrust

Jumping jacks, pushups

Medicine ball side toss, medicine ball slam

As you get the hang of the above exercise, start the next:

Hurricane Workouts

This is essentially a workout protocol that entails lifting weights and interval training. We have three groups of exercises, called rounds in this type of workouts. Each round has an exercise that increases your heart rate, and a set of other exercises in between.

This design will allow you to keep your heart rate up throughout the workout (and burn significant amounts of calories) that typically lasts 16-22 minutes. Hurricane workouts have five levels and each one is an increased challenge. I have however prepared for you a sample routine you will work with below.

Note: This will require you to be more fit- if fit enough though, you can begin with this:

Warm up for the workout. For all rounds, do one set of each exercise and move on to the next exercise. Finish the whole round thrice before you move to the next round.

First round: Run on a treadmill at 10% incline, 10.5 mph for 25 seconds. Do a kettlebell Turkish getup about 4 times on each side of your body then 10 chin-ups.

Repeat this sequence thrice.

Second round: Run on a treadmill at a 10% incline, 11 mph for 25 seconds. Do 10 dips and a barbell rollout, 15 reps.

Repeat this process thrice.

Third round: Run on a treadmill at a 10% incline, 11.5 mph for 25 seconds. Perform the G.I row, 10 reps. Do the knee grab, 20 reps.

Repeat three times.

I need your help...

Thank you for buying this book!

I hope this book was able to help you to know more about the Negative Calorie Diet and how you can burn fat and lose weight with this diet, the next step is to put what you have learned into practice and actually adopt the diet if you want to see those pounds coming off.

Finally, if you enjoyed this book, then I'd like to ask you for a favor, would you be kind enough to leave a review for this book on Amazon? It'd be greatly appreciated!

I want to reach as many people as I can with this book, and more reviews will help me accomplish that!

If you have any questions or problems, please contact us: hello@freedomdestination.com

Thank you and good luck!

20 Easy And Fast Diet Tips For Losing Weight

An Easy-To-Follow Weight Loss Guide

LELA GIBSON

INTRODUCTION

I want to thank you and congratulate you for buying the book, *"20 Easy and Fast Diet Tips for Losing Weight"*.

This book has actionable information on how to lose weight and live a much healthier life.

Maintaining a healthy weight is an important part of living a long and healthy life. If you are struggling with obesity, you know better than anyone that being overweight affects your social life.

Inasmuch as many try to hide it, the truth is that it is usually very difficult to manage interpersonal relationships. You might be the all-confident type of person who seems not to care what others say or think about your weight or lifestyle but the truth is that many aspects of your life (which you are well aware of) are not going on right because you are carrying some excess weight.

While it is good to be confident and love yourself as much as possible, we have to note that the risks and negative effects of being overweight pose a real threat to your emotional and physical well-being. We could spend a whole day discussing about the diseases such as heart disease and stroke that breed from increases in weight, and perhaps another to discuss further about the mental/emotional conditions that may arise as well. Overall, the truth is that whether you consider yourself a BBW or whatever fond name you give yourself, if you desire to live a long and healthy life, you need to do something about losing that excess weight.

This book discusses 20 of the best ways to lose weight so that you live better in many aspects including being more comfortable and thriving in interpersonal relationships, maintaining a good mental and physical health, and living a more positive life.

Thanks again for buying this book. I hope you enjoy it!

CONTENTS

Introduction   50

Why You Need To Lose Weight   54

20 Easy and Fast Diet Tips for Losing Weight   61

Take Advantage of Water

1: Drink Water throughout the Day   63

2: Always Drink a Glass of Water before Every Meal   64

Check Your Food Intake

3: Eat the Right Foods   65

4: Avoid Particular Foods   68

5: Eat Breakfast   70

Shop Smart

6: Pay Cash at the Store   71

7: Do Not Underestimate the Power of the List   72

8: Start With the Local Section   73

Tune in When You Eat

9: Pay Attention and Avoid Distractions While Eating   74

10: Mix Things and Stop When You Are Full   75

Alter Your Environment

11: Clear 'Em All!   76

12: Let Your Environment Remind You That You   77
Are Changed

13: Work With Pictures   79

Eat Less

14: Maintain a Food Diary   80

15: Eat Your Meals Close To Mirrors   82

16: Commit To Cooking Your Own Food/Don't Buy   83
Prepared Food

17: Love Blue, Adopt Blue   85

18: Get a Ribbon   86

Reward Yourself

19: Adopt Snacks That Burn Fat!   87

20: Fire up Your Meals   90

Conclusion   91

Preview Of '20 Easy And Fast Diet Tips For Losing   92
Weight – An Easy-To-Follow Weight Loss Guide: '

Check Out My Other Books   99

Bonus: Subscribe To The Free Weight Loss Report   105

Before we start learning about the strategies you can use to lose weight, let's start by highlighting some of the benefits that will come as a result of shedding those extra pounds just to give you extra motivation to want to do something NOW.

Why You Need To Lose Weight

Healthy weight loss has over one hundred benefits; these include emotional and physical benefits. I will dedicate this section to discussing the health benefits that many people (and weight loss/health books) do not pay enough attention to.

1: You Avoid Pre-Diabetes or Type 2 Diabetes

Pre-diabetes/high blood glucose is a condition that develops when the blood sugar levels in your blood move past normal ranges but not enough to qualify as diabetes. When your body stops consistently producing insulin sufficient to meet your body's needs, or the amount produced does not work properly, type 2 diabetes is likely to develop. Being pre-diabetic places you at a very high risk of developing type 2 diabetes.

Being obese or overweight is a proven leading risk factor for type 2 diabetes because carrying excess weight typically makes it hard for cells to respond to insulin, and since the additional fat acts as an insulating layer, it makes it more difficult for the sugar to enter the cells, which results in more circulating blood sugar levels.

Nonetheless, if you are already a pre-diabetic, you can prevent the progression to diabetes by shedding some weight (to reduce the insulating layer on cells so that they respond more to insulin) and trying to maintain a healthy weight.

2: You Keep Your Heart Healthy

When it comes to heart disease, some of the key risk factors are high cholesterol and high blood pressure. Research shows that:

1. Excessive accumulation of body fat makes your body release particular chemicals that occur naturally into the bloodstream, which increases blood pressure, and

2. Being overweight makes the liver produce too much amounts of Low density Lipoprotein (LDL) also called cholesterol. LDL tends to be sticky and gathers in the walls of blood vessels, which causes the narrowing of arteries, a condition called atherosclerosis, which increases your risk of strokes and heart attack.

When you lose weight, your blood pressure often reduces and the liver naturally reduces the amount of LDL it produces.

Royal Adelaide Hospital conducted a research on cardiovascular improvements with respect to a special weight loss program. Their results showed a decrease of cholesterol by 12%, a 10% decrease of LDL, a 5% decrease in diastolic blood pressure, and an 8% decrease in systolic blood pressure.

3: Improved Sleep (and Possible Treatment of Sleep Apnea)

One of the most prominent benefits of losing weight is improved sleep. When you gain excess weight, you gather more soft tissues in the neck; this intensifies the incidence of snoring.

NOTE: Snoring is a result of constricted airways, which obstructs air movement.

Snoring can be a symptom of sleep apnea, a possible life-threatening condition characterized by obstruction of breathing that requires the victim to wake up frequently from sleep to resume breathing.

As a victim of sleep apnea, you rarely remember anything about the episodes of waking many times a night to breathe but even so, this sleep and oxygen deprivation could easily lead to a weak immune system, high blood pressure, heart disease, memory problems, and sexual dysfunction.

When you lose weight, you reduce the amount of fatty tissue in the back of your throat, decrease snoring and the likelihood of the worsening of your health- as aforementioned. You encourage better sleep quality and reduce the risk of developing sleep apnea.

4: Better Joints (Mobile and Pain-Free)

Osteoarthritis (OA) is one of the most common joint disorders. It causes the tissues that protect the joints (cartilage and bone) to wear away. Consequently, the joints become tender and swollen, thus making movement very painful.

When you are overweight, you add to the load placed on the joints that bear the weight such as hips and knees.

NOTE: When you walk, you exert a force of approximately 3-6 times your entire body weight across the knee (read more on this page (check the discussion section) or here), so adding about 10 kg of weight does increase the force on the knees, which is equal to carrying 30-60 kgs[2] extra.

Therefore, a loss of merely 5% of your body weight could reduce the amount of stress placed on the knees, lower back, and hips, and reduce the pain (remember that losing 5kgs is equal to relieving a force of 15-30kgs[2] on the knees). According to doctors, a 10% loss of bodyweight has presented a 28% improvement in knee osteoarthritis symptoms.

5: Improved Fertility

There is epidemiological evidence that proves being obese has negative effects on reproduction. There has not been clarity in the mechanisms underlying the relationship between infertility and obesity but research studies suggest that excess body can lead to a serious offset in the metabolism of sex hormones that produce menstrual disruption and consequently, subfertility.

Moreover, when you are pregnant and overweight, you a more likely to miscarry and (or) develop other medical complications, and in particular, gestational diabetes, pregnancy induced hypertension, thromboembolism, and preeclampsia. There are reports to show that deliveries in obese women show increased rates of labor induction, caesarian section, and problematic labor caused by increased size of the unborn baby.

Additionally, experts report that a baby of an overweight woman is more likely to require more medical attention (admission to neonatal intensive care) and develop congenital defects such as cardiac and neural tube problems.

Moreover, obese individuals are more likely to experience birth related injuries and the likelihood of giving birth to babies with large birth weights, which puts them at risk of birth trauma and a possibility of childhood and probably lifelong obesity. Reducing weight in this case could help you and your baby avoid all these health problems.

Emotional Weight Loss Benefits

The negativity usually around overweight people affects your self-esteem and confidence. Naturally, when you are carrying some excess weight, you will worry about how other people see you and become overly anxious in particular situations. This affects many aspects of your life including your job interactions and performance, school, and your life at home (in the neighborhood).

Losing weight will help you gain confidence and increase your self-worth and self-love; losing weight normally makes you cheerful and as a result, your relationships with other people improve. Most of your fears and anxieties related to being overweight disappear and in general, you live a better life.

Once you regain your confidence, you feel in control. This becomes the status quo once you become comfortable with your new weight. Once you lose the weight, you are more comfortable when making food related decisions.

You also feel and become more honest when you interact with others and can better articulate your thoughts and feelings. You will no longer hold back since you are more self-possessed about your appearance and health.

Now that you know some of the benefits you stand to gain from losing weight, let us discuss the various effortless ways to lose weight.

20 Easy and Fast Diet Tips for Losing Weight

This book will be very straightforward with you: when we say easy, we do not mean that the weight will magically vanish when you implement the tips and strategies listed here. What we do mean, however, is that if you consistently practice what we preach here (the tips are strategies we shall discuss are easy to adopt into your everyday routine), you shall lose weight no doubt.

Let's begin.

Take Advantage of Water

In your effort to lose weight, water can be one of your strongest weapons. Not only does water boost metabolism, it suppresses your appetite and helps you lose water weight. Yes, drinking water makes you lose water that your body retains to support itself when you do not drink enough.

Water is normally one of the things your kidneys excrete under normal circumstances. However, when you do not drink enough water, your body stores as much of it as it can get (as though there is a famine) to reuse, which makes you look fat and bloated. Drinking water has more benefits in regards to weight loss than many people know!

Nonetheless, I know that taking the recommended 8-10 glasses each day can be rather difficult. With the tips I'm going to discuss shortly and determination, you will lose weight faster than you would ever think.

1: *Drink Water throughout the Day*

Water helps you remain full for longer without having to consume anything else (which is usually high calorie beverages like juice, milk [1 cup of 244g typically contains 103 calories], some teas, plus snacks), which would make you add weight.

Drinking water throughout the day can potentially save you a significant number of calories.

1. Don't like plain water? Try flavored water. Many stores stock calorie-free flavor packets that can give you a more tasty water experience. You can also add flavor to your water by using various foods. Fruits such as watermelon and vegetables such as cucumber tend to change the taste of water. Thus, instead of having that bland taste that is easy to hate, you'll have something better to look forward to.

2. Use a reminder: If you are serious about losing weight, set an alarm to remind you to drink water at particular times during the day. An alarm (especially a loud one) essentially pushes you to drink water when you do not feel like it. With time, it becomes a habit to drink water more regularly.

3. Keep more water close by. Keep a refillable bottle in your office, bedroom, and your bag and walk with it most of the time.

4. Replace most sweetened beverages with water. Most sweetened drinks contain sugars your body tends to convert to fat. As I said, calories are very prevalent in such drinks too.

2: Always Drink a Glass of Water before You Eat

The feeling of being full will push you into eating less, which is also another contributory way to lose weight since you end up consuming less calories for better weight loss results.

If you want much better results, make it a habit to drink a glass of water before, during, and after the meal. Water also aids digestion, which quickens weight loss. The nutrients you will consume will break down better and absorbed quickly, something your body needs to remain healthy especially as you incorporate different ways to lose weight (some of them such as fasting might threaten to leave you under-nourished) so your body has to learn to take up fewer nutrients faster.

Check Your Food Intake

You have gained weight because you have given yourself an all-access-pass to eating to your heart's content. That has to change. Do –

3: Eat the Right Foods

What you eat determines how much you store or lose; you therefore ought to take more care about what you eat. The following foods have proven to help people lose weight in their own special way:

Eggs

The misconception has always been that only the white part of the egg is beneficial. That is not true. The whole egg is nutritious, and the yolk only holds half the protein. The egg proteins stimulate the release of glucagon, a hormone that helps burn fat and is actually one of the best foods to aid in getting rid of belly fat.

Eggs are some of the foods we cannot eat in excess because they get us full quick and keep us full for longer (note that staying full is vital in any weight loss program).

Almond Butter and Raw Almonds

We all know that peanut butter is choke full of protein and that almonds are some of the best quality nuts around which are rich in vitamin E. This nutrient is actually an antioxidant that is very useful in offsetting free-radical damage.

Besides being good for your skin and hair, almonds contain Vitamin B2 and magnesium that helps calm the nerves and combat stress. Typically, when you feel stressed, the body releases a hormone called cortisol into the blood stream, and then through a series of events in the body, causes weight gain. Vitamin B2 in particular also helps boost your energy levels.

Chia Seeds

Chia seeds are rich in calcium, iron, and omega-3 fatty acids. They aid weight loss because they absorb sugar and thus contribute greatly to stabilizing your body sugar levels. Since they contain a lot of fiber, these small seeds can hold about twenty times their entire weight in water, and when they mix with liquid, they absorb as much as possible.

All you need to do in this case is add them to your oatmeal, or just place them in a bowl containing unsweetened chocolate almond milk. You can also eat them as 'chia water'. Just soak 40 grams of chia seeds in a liter of water for 25 minutes.

Fruits and Vegetables

We cannot talk about losing weight without mentioning fruits and veggies. Fruits and veggiesaid in weight loss because they are low in calories and high in numerous important nutrients such as vitamins and fiber.

Practically, fruits and vegetables fill you up without loading you up with calories and fat. When your stomach is full from low calorie food, it reduces your chances of binging on other 'bad' foods.

Research suggests that plant-based foods help in the control of food cravings and overeating. As you select your fruits and vegetables, it would be wise to remember that not all fruits and vegetables are equal. Some are healthier than others are and others are high in carbohydrates.

If you frequently indulge in fruits and vegetables that are high in carbs, you'll end up sabotaging your weight loss efforts. This is especially so if you consume such foods as juices or smoothies.

4: Avoid Particular Foods

Avoid foods that fall into the following categories:

Any Snack That Only Contains Carbohydrates

Snacks such as bread, crackers, and rice cakes are pure carbs. When you eat them, your body converts them to simple sugars and deposits them into your bloodstream. This sugar rush makes your body produce more insulin to help body absorb the sugar immediately.

The problem is that you end up with low blood sugar and the same feelings of hunger that led you to snack in the first place. You then find yourself reaching for 'quick' sugary foods to satisfy your craving for instant energy.

Do not forget that once in your body, this sugar converts into fat when in excess, which makes things worse. This is not limited to snacks alone, even potatoes are not entirely good. If you do not exercise often, potatoes should only make an occasional appearance in your food list. Just like French fries, venerable baked potato increase the levels of blood sugar and insulin quicker and to higher levels far much more than the same amount of calories from table sugar. French fries might be worse because they come with an added blast of fat.

The best way to avoid eating the wrong type of snacks is to ensure that you keep low calorie snacks handy. When you plan for cravings beforehand, you will be better prepared to deal with them successfully.

Frozen Foods

Food manufacturers usually fill frozen foods with sodium to act as a natural preservative in order to make fresh ingredients last longer in your freezer. Sodium makes you retain water, which tends to bloat you up, which becomes a problem to any weight loss program because it makes you look fat even when you have lost weight.

Very Little Fat

Contrary to what mainstream media has led us into believing, fat-restricted diets do not directly translate into reduced body fat. The truth is that embracing a bit more fat could help you much more lose weight.

There are many reasons why low-fat diets make you gain weight (and thus thwart your weight loss efforts). One of the most prominent reasons is that such diets have negative effects on hormones called adipokines released specifically from your fat cells. Adiponectin is one such hormone that burns fat by enhancing your metabolism and boosting the rates at which your body breaks down fat, controlling your appetite. Lower-fat diets reduce the levels of adiponectin.

NOTE: Be careful here. There are bad and good fats. I would recommend you only go for monounsaturated fats such as avocados, natural peanut butter, olives, and nuts, and polyunsaturated fats such as walnuts, soymilk and sesame, flux, pumpkin, and sunflower seeds.

5: Eat Breakfast

Numerous studies have discovered that *not skipping breakfast* is one of the most vital ways to lose weight quickly.

When you skip breakfast, your blood sugar drops. You thus become hungry and have less energy. What do you do? You impulsively snack – usually on high sugar snacks or fast foods, or (and) eat extra servings at lunch, and perhaps at dinner.

One 2005 study found that people who skip breakfast often find ways to compensate later during the day with more refined carbohydrates and unhealthy fats, with fewer green vegetables and fruits. When you eat enough breakfast, your body feels nourished and satisfied, which decreases the chances that you will overeat during the day.

You can create time for breakfast by doing some other things before you go to bed. For example, you can arrange your clothes for the day and organize your home before going to bed. This way, when you wake up, you will have fewer things to do and a lot of time to eat breakfast.

Shop Smart

Losing weight is a process that has to include what you pick from the stores. Unfortunately, it can be difficult to pick the right (healthy) foods that aid weight loss. The tips below have you covered in this regard.

6: Pay Cash at the Store

Based on research, consumers who buy things with actual cold, hard cash tend to spend less and make wiser decisions in what they buy than their counterparts who pay with plastic.

Parting with your actual physical hard-earned cash creates some sort of 'pain of payment' that lessens the *enjoyment of consumption.* This logic applies to your shopping habits at the grocery store. Those who use cash make better food choices while at the grocery store than those who pay with plastic.

The study clearly states that when consumers come across vice things such as pies, cookies, and cakes, the emotive imagery, and the desire associated with it stimulates impulsive purchase decisions. The pain of payment is therefore vital in curbing the impulsive responses.

7: *Do Not Underestimate the Power of the List*

According to a new study, having a shopping list could be the one reason you do not require expensive workouts and fasting programs.

During the study, those who reported to having used a list when shopping had a much healthier weight compared to those who did not, and the same replicated itself even in neighborhoods that had various obstacles to healthy eating.

A different study clearly shows that sticking to a list when you shop is a vital factor in weight loss. The thing is, when you have a list, you can counteract many influences that are always shouting at us at the store, urging you not to necessarily go for healthy food options.

As you make your list, you should start with the 'must-haves' items. These are healthy food items that you need to purchase before you even think of buying something else. If you make it a habit to buy such items, you will find that you will not have a lot of cash to spend on unhealthy junk food, and that is a good thing.

8: Start With the Local Section

Each time you visit the store, make it a habit to start at the local produce section, or look out for labels indicating that the veggies and fruits are local. This is a good way to get the season's peak picks and still pay less while buying something you may not always eat. Moreover, even if you do not find a label indicated organic – it is (often) just too costly for local farmers to get certified – fresh is always good.

Tune in When You Eat

The world in which we live has become increasingly fast-paced and our eating has become mindless. We are always eating on the run, while watching the TV, at the desk while working ...all of which causes us to eat a lot more than we need. In order to practice mindful eating, do the following:

9: Pay Attention and Avoid Distractions While Eating

You need to eat slowly while savoring the texture and smells of your food. Just like a simple eating meditation, do not let your mind wander. When it does, gently bring it back to your food and its tastes.

Again, you need to avoid distractions: do not eat while doing something else such as driving, writing, watching TV, or completing a project. It is not hard to overeat if, as you do so, you engage in other things.

You should also avoid eating from a bowl or serving from a serving dish especially when you're distracted. If you consume food when it is in a large container, you'll continue serving yourself without paying much attention to how many calories you are consuming. You need to serve your food in a plate and refrain from taking 'seconds' or 'thirds'. Also remember that you don't have to finish everything on your plate if you're full. You can always use leftovers later when preparing other meals.

10: Mix Things and Stop When You Are Full

It is important to mix things up in order to focus on the eating experience. You can use chopsticks rather than the fork or hold everything with the other hand; this way, you will stay focused.

Do not continue eating when you feel full. Eating mindfully helps you easily know when you are full. You should also not feel obligated to leave your plate empty.

Alter Your Environment

Changing your environment is a good reinforcement to ensure you stay committed to your weight loss efforts. Why is this important? Well, it is important because it makes the change you have decided to bring into your life appear more real and practical. It requires a strong and determined heart though; but only requires the following:

11: Clear 'Em All!

Clean out your fridge, cupboard, pantry, and the kitchen shelves. Go to the bedroom and do the same to all shelves and hiding spots for food. At your workplace, clear your drawers of any junk foods kept there. Ideally, remove all junk foods from all the places you spend time in because when they are in your immediate environment, they can easily sabotage your success.

Perhaps you thought the junk was good to keep you busy when you are bored or hungry but you are too busy to go out for lunch. You can easily replace them with fruits if you are addicted to biting on something every so often.

You can occasionally eat junk food, but do not stock it.

12: *Let Your Environment Remind You That You Are Changed*

You have decided to change your diet completely. You have decided to stay committed to the course of losing weight no matter what. Let your environment be a constant reminder that you are indeed new; that you will no longer indulge in bad eating habits and will instead adopt the healthy ones as we have discussed so far- now change it!

Rearrange your bedroom, living room, and any other area of your house where you spend a lot of your time in – perhaps including your office. Switch the chairs, move the couch to the other side, change the location of your TV.

Go to your bedroom and change the bed to the other side of the room, get your alarm clock onto the other dresser- or across the room so that when you wake up and roll over to hit snooze, you realize it is not there and you have to walk across the room. This will be an instant reminder of the new you.

The idea is to disrupt your previous routine and create new habits. Make no mistake. Eating unhealthy foods is a habit. It is a bad habit that starts with you purchasing such foods. It is followed by you forming associations that enable the bad habit. For example, you may enjoy eating pizza and drinking soda during 'movie night'. That is a habit. In order to break one habit, you have to create a new habit that will be better for you as far as losing weight is concerned. In this case, you can create the habit of having a healthy meal before you see your movie and drinking water during the movie.

You can create other new habits. You can make it a habit to get up whenever you want to change the television channel. It is a small thing but it will get your heart pumping. You can make it a habit to lockdown the kitchen for the night. This will prevent you from late night snacking and it will help you lose weight. You can also create a habit of walking around the house. For example, when setting the table, instead of carrying many things at once, you can carry one or two items at a time so that you can walk for longer. These little changes will become part of your new routine and they will help you to lose weight.

13: Work With Pictures

Pictures, Pictures, Pictures: have many of them; they always work. What motivates you? Is it walking confidently in the streets as you used to? Having a great body, or perhaps being able to engage in particular fun (game) activities with friends or your kids?

Whatever is driving you to lose weight, hang many different pictures that describe it all over the place: In your bedroom, on the fridge door, above the dressing mirror, in the car's dashboard...everywhere! Let them keep your eyes on the prize.

Eat Less

To lose weight, sometimes the general advice comes in handy: *eat less.* Nevertheless, like other tips we have thus far discussed, eating less can be hard when you are already used to eating large potions and eating many times during the day. Nonetheless, I will make it simple: you just need to adjust a few things and adopt a few others such as the following:

14: Maintain a Food Diary

Studies have discovered that people who keep food diaries always end up eating 15% less, and more healthier foods. In this regard, you need to watch out for the weekends. A study conducted by the University of North Carolina discovered that people tend to eat an extra 115 calories per day during the weekends – especially from alcohol and fat.

Since your focus is on losing weight, keeping a food diary should be easy while the benefits are instantaneous. The diary essentially builds your awareness of what you eat, how much and why you are eating it, something that helps you cut down on mindless eating.

Further, the diary will help you identify foods you need to reduce or add against the ideal 'weight loss food list' (whose basic scheme and contents you have a rough idea of already – I hope) as you monitor your intake progress.

You don't have to keep a boring food diary showing only what foods you've eaten. You can make it more interesting by stating how the food made you feel. You can even go ahead to compare recipes and criticize others. You can also note down which oils, herbs and spices go well with which foods. The idea is to take the whole experience like a project or an adventure that will require accounting at the end of it. This will give you the motivation you need to see it through.

15: Eat Your Meals Close To Mirrors

Many studies have tried to investigate this possibility and most of them have presented positive results. One of the most popular studies found that eating right in front of a mirror reduced how much people actually ate by almost one-third.

The main argument is that looking yourself in the eye does reflect back some of your own inner principles, standards, and goals, and reminds you why you are changing your eating habits in the first place. It is unbelievable, but true.

The idea is so good that it also works for people who do not necessarily have weight loss goals:

The University of Florida conducted a research that used 185 student participants asked to select between a chocolate cake and a serving of fruit salad. They ate in two rooms- one had a mirror and the other did not.

The students with the chocolate cake inside a room with mirrors reported to having found the cake less tasty, compared to their counterparts who ate the cake inside a room without a mirror. The fruit salad group did not report any change in the food's taste.

16: Commit To Cooking Your Own Food/Don't Buy Prepared Food

This may sound like an oversimplification but it is true: *the less you cook, the more you gain weight.* According to a recent report by john Hopkins University, home cooking is one of the best ways to lose weight and maintain a healthy weight.

The report's rationale is that folks who prepare their own dinners most nights have a tendency of consuming significantly less sugar, calories, and unhealthy fat than people who love eating out. According to the report, at-home chefs in particular consume about 140 less calories per day, which could add up to a couple of pounds of extra weight in a short period.

People who cook their own food cut back on sugar and unhealthy fat in similar proportions.

NOTE: The people the study talks about do not necessarily seek to lose weight. You can thus imagine how much healthier people who are looking to lose weight are bound to be when they cook for themselves.

When you resolve to cook for yourself, this general rule might come in handy: find a less-sugar version of the same type of food you think contains a lot of sugar, or sugar free varieties such as salad dressing, mayonnaise, and ketchup.

Avoid hydrogenated foods and look for not less than two grams of fiber for every 100 calories in all grain products. I hope you know that a shorter list of ingredients is better because it means less empty calories and flavor enhancers.

Another good thing about cooking for yourself is that you can experiment with different foods. You can make healthier substitutions to items called for in a recipe and you can try out various recipes to keep things interesting.

17: Love Blue, Adopt Blue

It is all about simple color psychology.

Some colors represent different meanings and elicit different feelings. For instance, red depicts intense emotion, and green is for luck and stress relief. Blue on the other hand has a calming effect, increases productivity, and has been strongly supported by studies to suppress appetite. There are not so many foods out there with this color, are there? Think about how it would make you feel to see blue in or on food.

Many diets recommend the use of this color and there are some recommended ways to use it for weight loss:

1. Eat all your food on a blue plate.

2. Install a blue light in your fridge

3. Install a blue light bulb in your dining room

4. If you are making food, you can also use dye into the food – just the thought of eating blue noodles or pancakes does not sit too well with many or the tummy.

Blue will make a great effect in making your appetite diminish, instantly.

18: Get a Ribbon

This tip is gaining fast popularity among the women. French women wear a thin ribbon (a bit above their waists) beneath their clothes. When they start eating and it gets tight, it means they have had too much. This is a good way to curb overeating because it can get very uncomfortable when you continue eating.

Reward Yourself

After remaining resolute as you pursue your weight loss goals, you can rewards yourself as follows:

19: *Adopt Snacks That Burn Fat!*

Adopt the use of the following snacks:

Power Berry Smoothie

Berries are great sources of antioxidants that protect body cells from damage that can lead to premature aging and disease. That is not all though, antioxidants are also associated with weight control.

A very recent research from the University of Florida reports that people who consume more antioxidants generally weigh less even when their calorie intake is not less.

More specifically, strawberries reduce blood sugar and insulin levels in your blood after you have had your meal. A key antioxidant in strawberries inhibits the activity of the enzyme responsible for breaking starch into glucose. This means less simple sugars will be released into your blood stream thus dropping blood sugar and of course, the corresponding insulin response.

For this reason, a power berry snack is one sweet way to weight loss and maintaining a healthy body.

What does it entail? Low-fat plain yogurt, soy protein powder and berries but you can add honey to make it sweeter and healthier.

Hot Chocolate

Stress is a leading cause of weight gain. Cocoa is also rich in antioxidants that target your levels of cortisol – cortisol is the stress hormone. This hormone makes your body cling to tummy fat. Hot chocolate is a good choice because it actually contains five times the amount of antioxidants found in black tea. It also contains compounds that lower the levels of insulin in the blood stream, which also keep the body from storing fat.

Best for last...

20: Fire up Your Meals

Eating does require a lot of energy, if you select the right foods. These foods will stimulate your body to burn more calories and in a special way, curb your appetite.

Chewy Foods: Vegetables, Whole Fruits, Lean Meats, and Nuts

These are active calories that make your body work off the fork. You can make the most of the chew factor by choosing the food in its whole state – go for a steak of tuna instead of canned tuna.

Here's the thing. You use up calories when you chew food. This translates to more weight loss. Thus, you should try to spend a few extra seconds on chewing your food. This action will also allow you to know when you are full because you will be taking some time off in between bites.

Warming Foods: Garlic, Peppers, Mustard, Cinnamon, Vinegar, Ginger and Cloves

Peppers in particular contain a chemical called capsaicin that gives it the burning sensation. It doubles the energy expenditure a few hours after eating (based on a study by UCLA). Even other mild peppers and ginger (that contain gingerol, a relative of capsaicin) and a blend of other similar spices contain compounds found to do away with up to 100 calories per day by affixing to nerve receptors and relaying fat burning signals to the brain.

Conclusion

There you have it; your top twenty diet tips to lose weight fast and without much hassle. As you select your favorites, make sure to cover at least every category for the most benefits.

Thank you again for buying this book!

I hope this book was able to help you to achieve your goal.

The next step is to take action.

Finally, if you enjoyed this book, then I'd like to ask you for a favor, would you be kind enough to leave a review for this book on Amazon? It'd be greatly appreciated!

I want to reach as many people as I can with this book, and more reviews will help me accomplish that!

If you have any questions or problems, please contact us: hello@freedomdestination.com

Thank you and good luck!

Preview Of 'Anti-Inflammatory Diet Guide '

Effects Of Inflammation

Inflammation is the biological response your body goes into when dealing with harmful stimuli such as irritants, pathogens or even damaged cells. It is a self-protection mechanism that allows your body to begin the healing process. The 'hotness' or 'inflammation' you feel after you cut yourself or injure yourself is the result of your body working hard to heal itself. But what happens when your body experiences 'too much' inflammation?

A little inflammation is not a bad thing. In fact, when it happens, you should rejoice in knowing that your body is working tirelessly to correct the situation. However, like most good things, inflammation can get out of hand. When this happens, you may experience various health complications such as:

Weight Gain

Every day, thousands of people try to lose weight to no avail. They complain that they've tried out various diets but somehow none seem to be working. If they do find something that works, sooner than later, they are back to gaining the weight they thought they'd lost. This is because they neglect to look into inflammation as the cause for their weight gain. Inflammation contributes to weight gain in various ways. These include:

- If inflammation happens in the brain, it interferes with the functioning of the hypothalamus and this in turn increases your appetite and slows down your metabolism. When this happens, you will be eating a lot but burning up less energy, which leads to weight gain.

- Gut inflammation leads to leptin and insulin resistance. Leptin is the satiety hormone that tells your brain when you have had enough. When suffering from leptin resistance, you just eat and eat some more before leptin can communicate that you have had enough, which leads to weight gain. Another thing that gut inflammation does is to increase intestinal permeability. When this happens, more toxins will be able to permeate your bloodstream. Usually toxins are stored in fat cells to remove them from circulation. The more toxins you have, the more the fat cells expand to accommodate the more toxins leading to weight gain.

- Inflammation in the endocrine system suppresses adrenal and thyroid function. One of the main functions of the adrenal gland is to burn fat. Therefore, when you suppress the functioning of the adrenal gland, you are unable to burn fat, as you should leading to weight gain.

As you have read, inflammation is bad for you if you want to maintain the ideal weight.

Metabolic Syndrome

Metabolic syndrome refers to a group/cluster of lifestyle-related diseases including cardiovascular disease and obesity. They are clustered together because all of these diseases are linked to metabolic dysfunction. Markers of metabolic dysfunction include:

- Central obesity – this is excessive tummy fat

- Hyperinsulinaemia – this refers to ongoing high levels of insulin

- Insulin resistance –your body loses sensitivity to insulin (you need more insulin to manage your blood sugar levels)

But the question is how these three factors are connected. Well, when on a diet high in carbohydrates, your blood sugar levels increase leading to high insulin levels to help blood cells absorb the glucose and thus manage your blood sugar levels. When you have high insulin levels, the production of cytokines (which are pro-inflammatory) increases and in turn this causes inflammation especially in predisposed persons. Once inflammation increases, it brings with it an increase in the production of free radicals. Free radicals affect cellular functions and one of those functions just happens to be insulin sensitivity. This is why chroni low-grade inflammation is linked to all three markers; that is, raised insulin levels, obesity and decreased insulin sensitivity.

Chronic Fatigue

Many people suffering from chronic fatigue have been told that the disease 'is all in their minds'. Fortunately, in recent years more researchers have began looking into the association of chronic fatigue and inflammation. This is mainly because the two possess many similar symptoms including muscular pain and tenderness, sore throat, joint pain, swollen lymph nodes and sore throat.

As you know, inflammation is the way your body reacts to foreign particles. When you have symptoms of inflammation, it is safe to say that your body is fighting something even if that something is not yet known. This is why researchers link an overactive immune system to chronic fatigue.

Another thing that associates chronic fatigue with inflammation is the lack of cortisol in patients suffering from chronic fatigue. Cortisol is known to suppress inflammation. Thus, if your body has a cortisol deficiency, it will not be able to suppress inflammation and this will worsen symptoms of chronic fatigue. A dietary change often helps people suffering from chronic fatigue.

Some types of arthritis

When you hear the name arthritis, you automatically associate it with pain. Well, it is no coincidence since arthritis refers to inflammation in joints. When your joints experience inflammation, you will feel pain. The types of arthritis that have been linked to inflammation include:

- Gouty arthritis

- Rheumatoid arthritis

- Psoriatic arthritis

- Systematic lupus erythematosus

When you suffer from these types of arthritis, you may experience inflammation symptoms such as redness, joint stiffness, swelling of the joints, pain in the joints and loss of joint function.

It is important to note that inflammation does not have to be painful for it to be present. This is because many organs in your body just don't have enough pain-sensitive areas for you to feel that inflammatory sensation. This means that you can suffer from chronic inflammation over time without knowing, only for you to experience the effects of inflammation.

It is also important to note that various things can cause inflammation including:

- Processed foods high in sugar and unhealthy fats

- Omega-6 fats (and not enough Omega-3 fatty acids)

- Sleep deprivation

- Chronic stress

- Smoking

- Pollution

- Environmental chemicals

- Lack of exercise

Thus, chances are, if you experience any of the above things, you may be suffering from inflammation whether or not you experience pain.

The first thing you should do once you notice that you suffer from inflammation is not to reach for drugs because drugs just address the symptoms and not the root cause but rather to make some lifestyle changes. This is because most of the causes of inflammation can be addressed by making lifestyle changes like exercising more, reducing exposure to pollutants, not smoking and dietary changes.

In this book, we will focus on addressing inflammation by adopting an anti-inflammatory diet. Let us learn more about anti-inflammatory diet in the next chapter.

Check out the rest of Anti-Inflammatory Diet Guide on Amazon, go to **http://amzn.to/2lDjVDU**

Check Out My Other Books

Below you'll find some of my other popular books that are popular on Amazon and Kindle as well

Alternatively, you can visit my author page on Amazon to see other work done by me.

Ketogenic Cookbook: Quick Low Calorie Ketogenic Crockpot Recipes with 7 Days Meal Plan

Freedom: How to Make Money Online and Become Financially Free by Creating Passive Income

Mediterranean Diet: Instant Pot Cookbook with Delicious Recipes

Alice the Superbug

Madison and Astrid's first magical journey

Intermittent Fasting: The Essential Beginners Guide for Women for Weight Loss

Chakra Healing: Chakra Healing and Karmic Awareness for Beginners

SEO 2017 for Growth: The Ultimate Guide to Learn Search Engine Optimization with Internet Marketing Tips

Psychology: How to Analyze People Using Human Psychological Techniques, Body Language Signals, Social Skills and Personality Types

Paleo Smoothies: Recipes to Energize and for Ultimate Health and Weight Loss

Belly Diet Smoothies: Delicious Smoothie Recipes to Flatten Your Belly, Improve Your Gut & Burn Fat

Keto Diet: Keto Diet Guide Cookbook for Beginners with Meal Plan and Simple, Delicious Recipes to Lose Weight and Look Good

Online Business from Scratch: The 9 Step Guide to Building a Profitable and Sustainable Online Business

Weight Loss: 20 Easy And Fast Diet Tips For Losing Weight - An Easy-To-Follow Weight Loss Guide

Ketogenic Cookbook: Ketogenic Cookbook for Beginners with 7 Days Meal Plan

Negative Calorie Diet: Cookbook & Guide Which Will Help You To Burn Body Fat, Lose Weight And Live Healthy

Negative Calorie Diet with Anti-Inflammatory Diet Guide

Make Money Online To Achieve Freedom

Negative Calorie Diet with Smart Fat Guide

Negative Calorie Diet & Clean Eating: Cookbook & Guide Which Will Help You To Burn Body Fat, Lose Weight And Live Healthy

Smart Fat: Cookbook with Fat Meals Which Help You to Lose Weight, Get Healthy and Improve Brain Function

Anti-Inflammatory Diet Guide: The Guide to Reduce Inflammation and Live a Healthy Life Without Pain

Essential Oils: The Young Living Book Guide of Natural Remedies for Beginners for Pets, For Dogs

Clean Eating: Cookbook and Guide to Restore Your Body's Natural Balance and Eat Healthy

Anti-Inflammatory Diet Guide: The Guide to Reduce Inflammation and Live a Healthy Life Without Pain

Dash Diet: Cookbook for Weight Loss with Action Plan and Easy Recipes

Air Fryer Cookbook: Quick, Healthy and Easy Low Carb Air Fryer Recipes

Psychology & Habits Of Highly Effective People Box Set

Leptin Resistance: Leptin Diet to Control Your Hormones, Get Permanent Weight Loss, Cure Obesity and Live Healthy

Negative Calorie Diet & Dash Diet Box Set

Negative Calorie Diet & Weight Loss Box Set

Habits of Highly Effective People: What Are the Habits of Successful People?

Slow Cooker: Cookbook with Slow Cooker Recipes

Weight Loss Cookbook: Meal Prep Cookbook for Weight Loss and Clean Eating

Weight Loss Cookbook: Mediterranean Diet for Lasting Weight Loss

Negative Calorie Diet & Dash Diet Box Set

Slow Cooker & Instant Pot Box Set

Children Books: Madison and Astrid's first magical journey & Alice the Superbug Box Set

Belly Diet: The Zero Belly Diet Step-By-Step Guide Which Helps You to Lose Your Belly and Enjoy Your Flat Belly

Weight Loss: 20 Easy and Fast Diet Tips for Losing Weight - An Easy-To-Follow Weight Loss Guide

Instant Pot: Instant Pot Pressure Cooker Cookbook with Easy and Healthy Recipes

Vegan Cookbook: Vegan Cookbook For Beginners, For Kids And For Teens For Diabetics With Pictures

Low Carb: Low Carb Diet Cookbook with Low Carb Keto Recipes for Batch Cooking

Ketogenic Cooking: Ketogenic Cooking With Your Instant Pot

Passive Income: Passive Income Tutorial with 7 Online Ideas to Generate Passive Income Streams for Beginners

Low Carb Diet: Low Carb Diet Recipes Cookbook for Beginners for Batch Cooking

Bonus: Subscribe To The Free Weight Loss Report

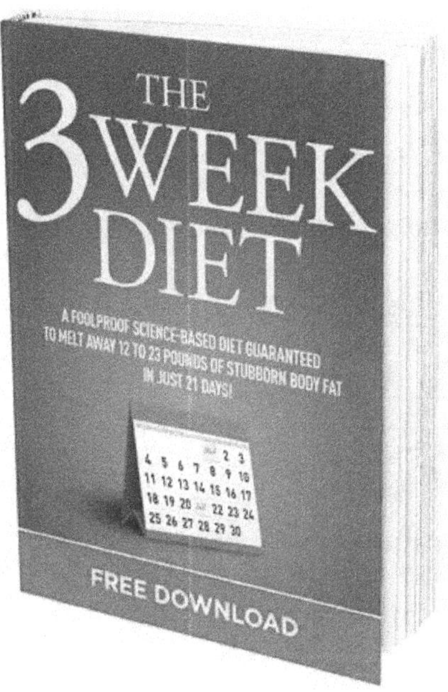

When you subscribe to Freedom Destination via email, you will get free access to an ebook. All you have to do is enter your email address to get instant access.

The Introduction Manual is more than just an introduction to the diet. Instead, it discusses the science behind how we gain and lose weight as well as what absolutely needs to be done to attack that stubborn body fat that, until now, has been so challenging to get rid of.

Here are the preview of what you'll get:

- Rapid Weight Loss

- How This System Works

- Why This Diet

- Why 3 Weeks?

- 21 Days To Make A Habit

- Fat Loss VS. Weight Loss

- Nutrients

- Protein, Fat, Carbohydrates

- The Food Pyramid And Obesity

- Fiber

- Metabolism

- How We Get Fat

- Triglycerides

- How To Get Thin

- Diet Overview

- Meal Frequency

- Water

- Diet Essentials

- Let's Get Started

To get instant access to these incredible ebook, go to: http://bit.ly/2tUb9cp

www.ingramcontent.com/pod-product-compliance
Lightning Source LLC
Chambersburg PA
CBHW072256260726
48658CB00001BA/411